McCoy has Food Allergies

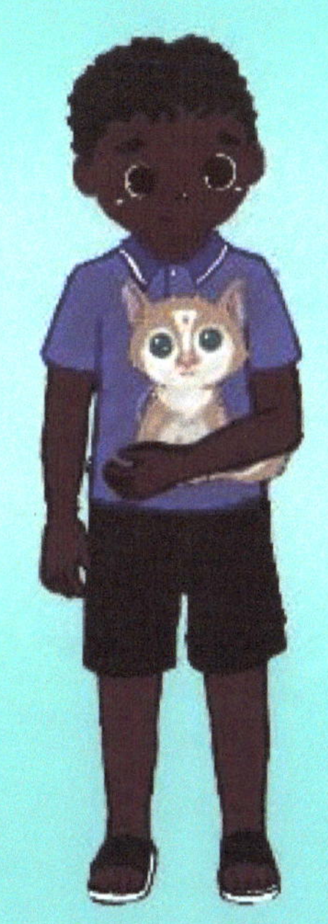

By W. G. McMillan

For
Emanuel McCoy
and
Eden Zane

McCoy has Food Allergies

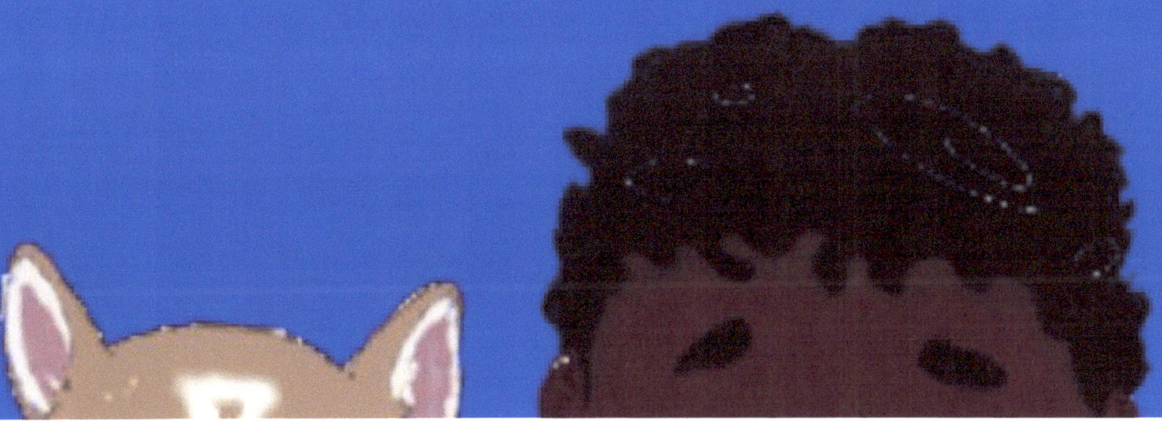

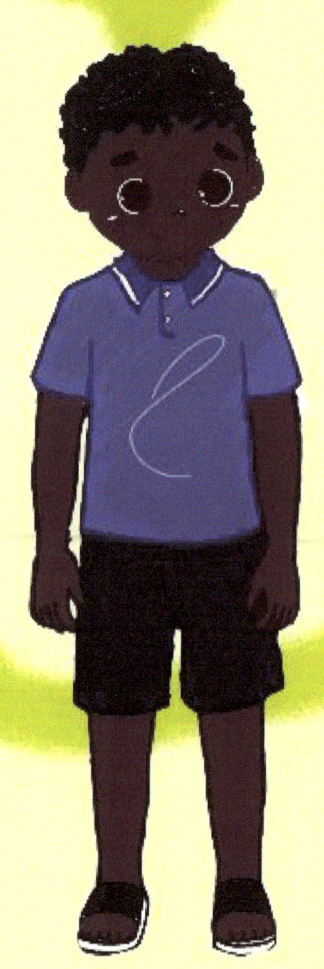

Hi, my name is McCoy and
I am four years old.

This is my dog Star.
She is my best friend.

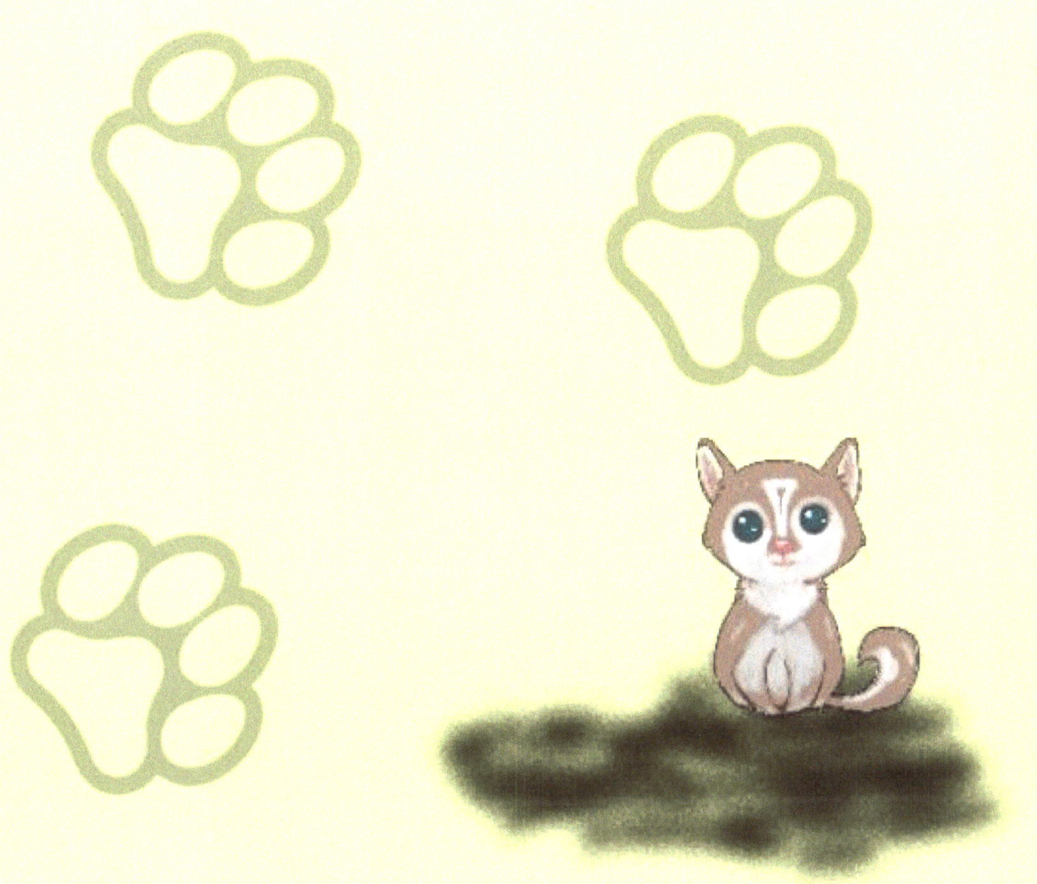

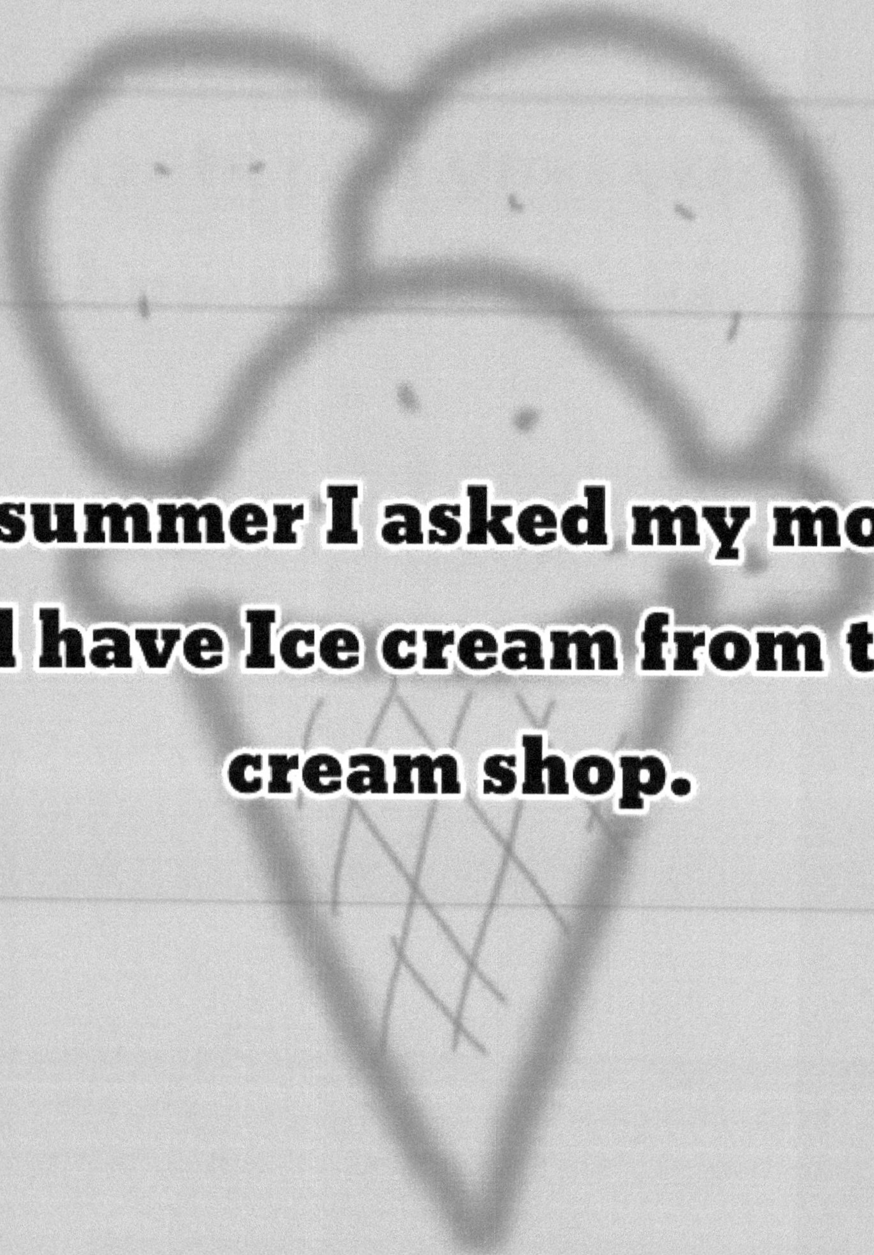

Last summer I asked my mom if I could have Ice cream from the ice cream shop.

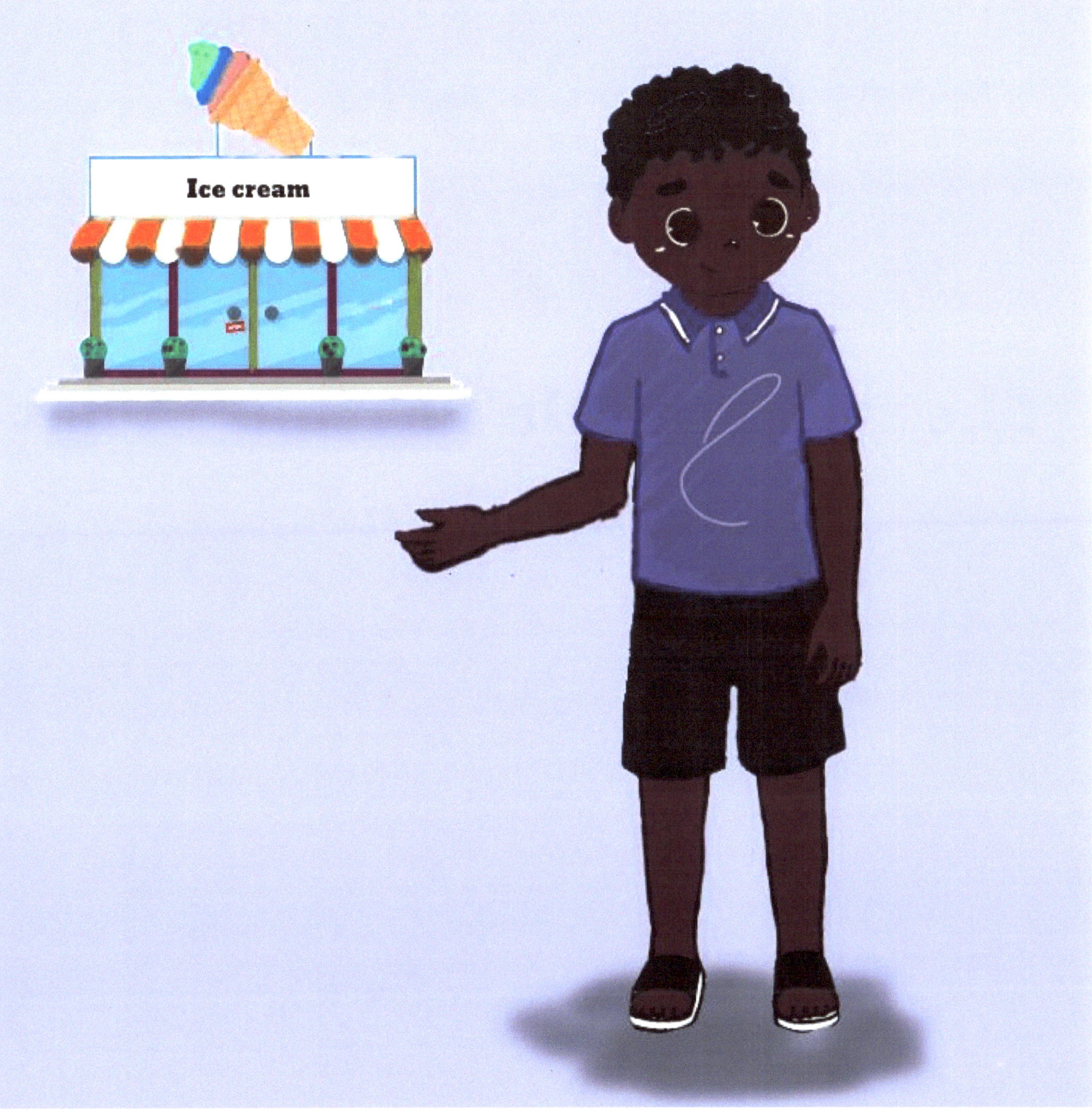
Ice cream

She said I couldn't because I have food allergies.

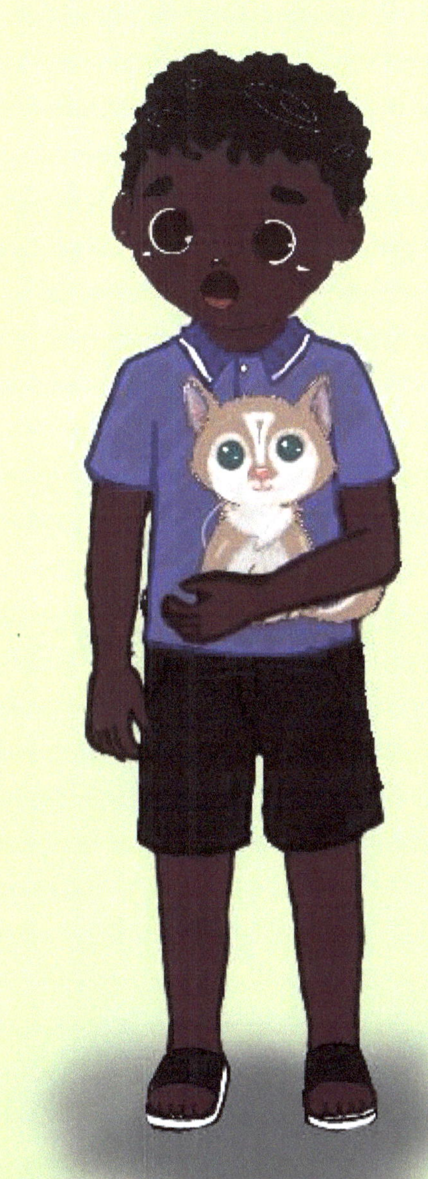

I was scared because I didn't know what food allergies were.

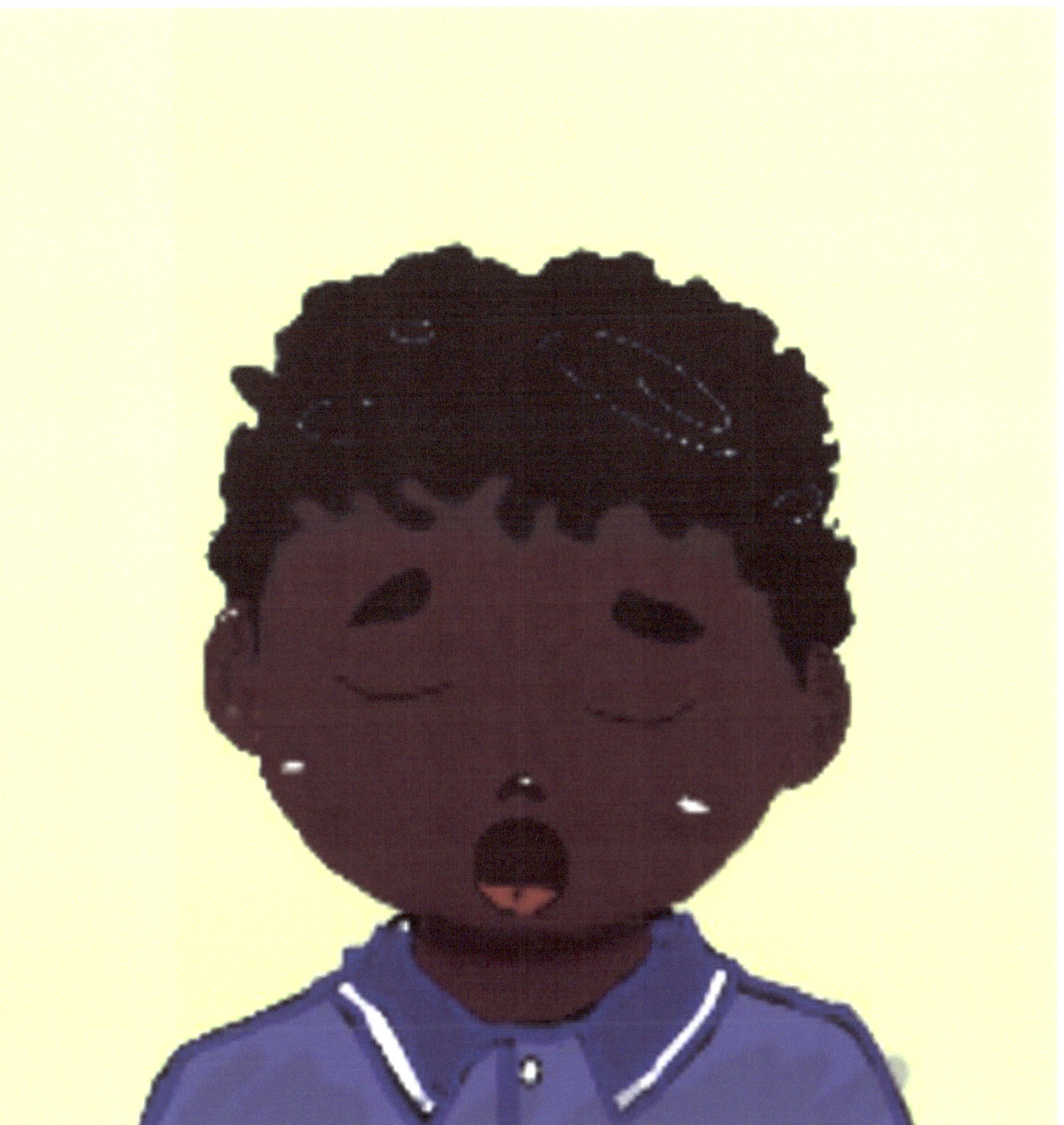

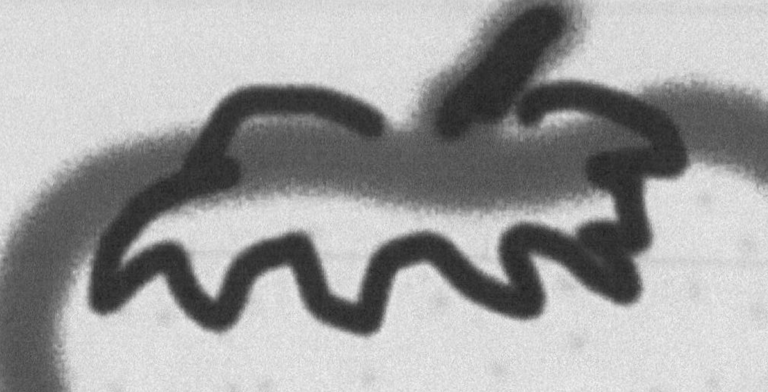

Mama told me that I can't eat some foods because they will make me sick.

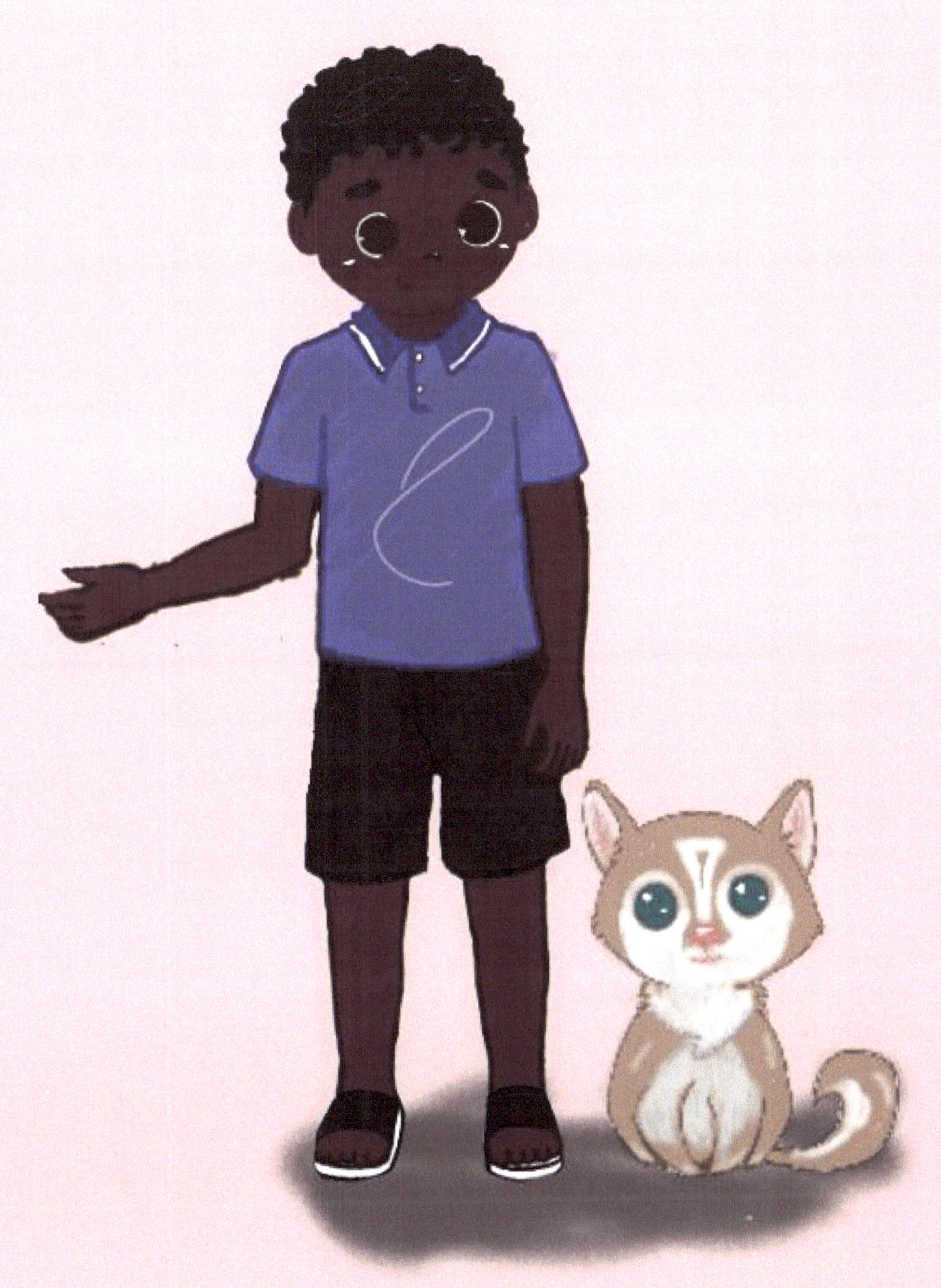

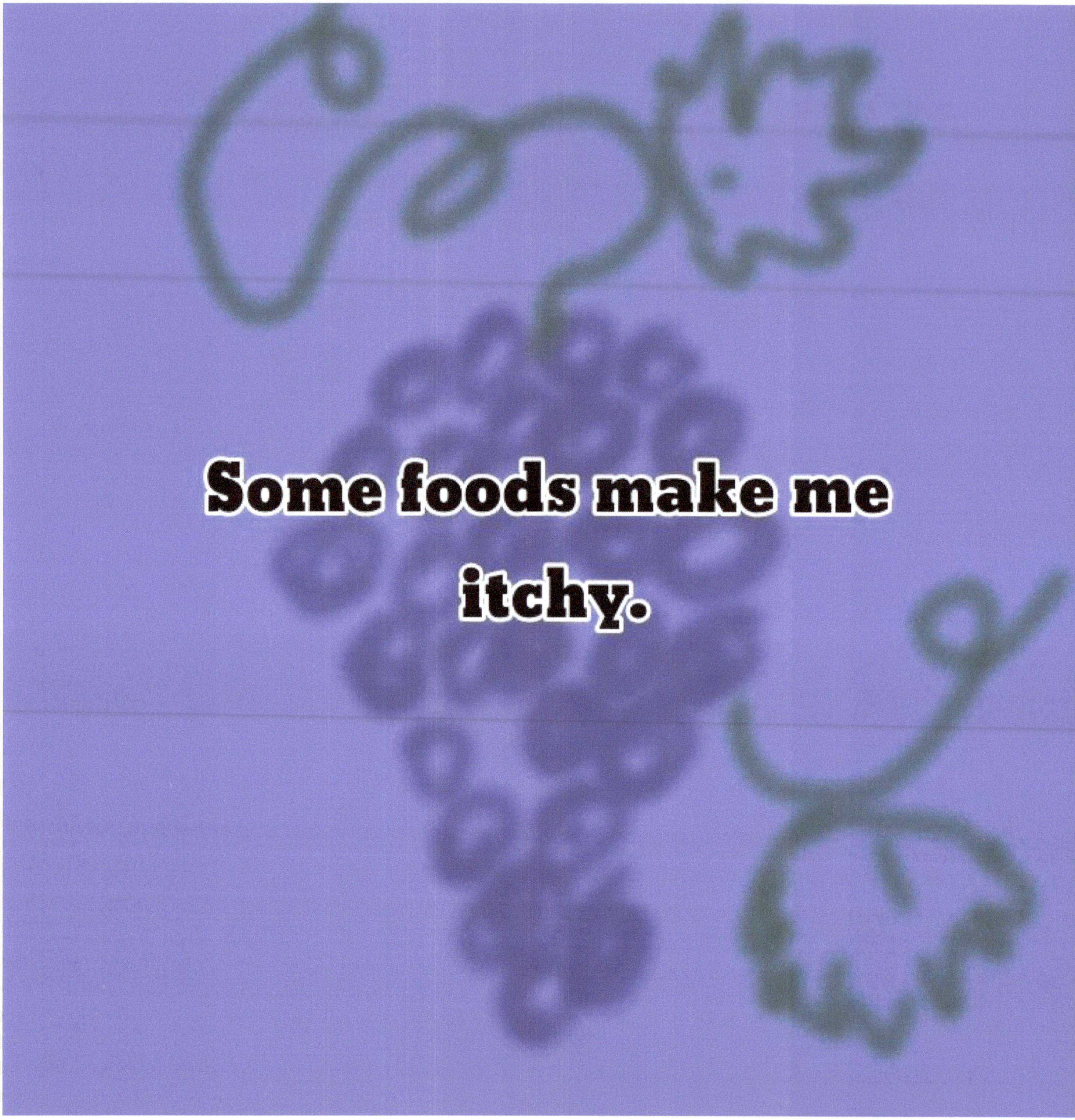

Some foods make me itchy.

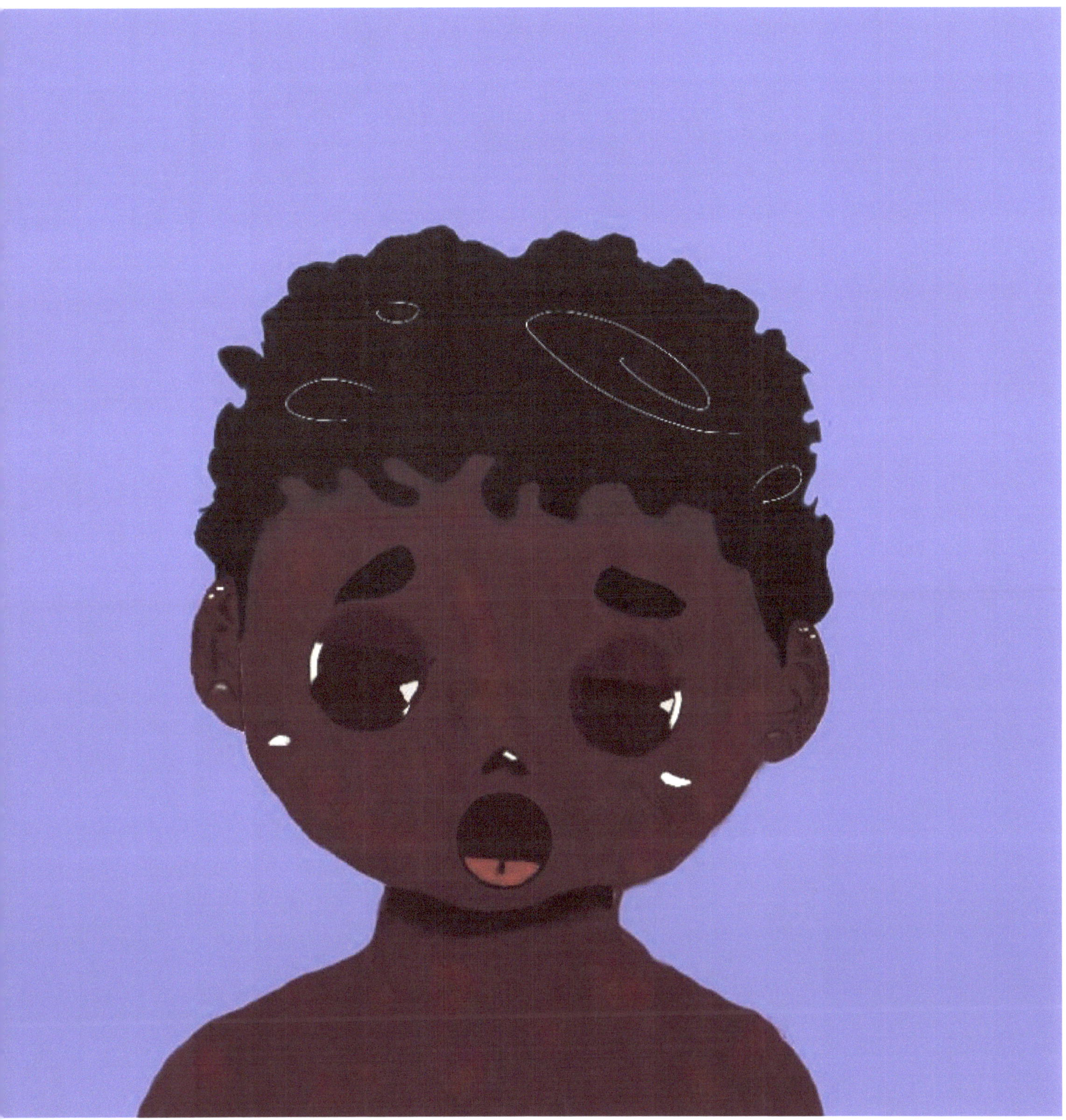

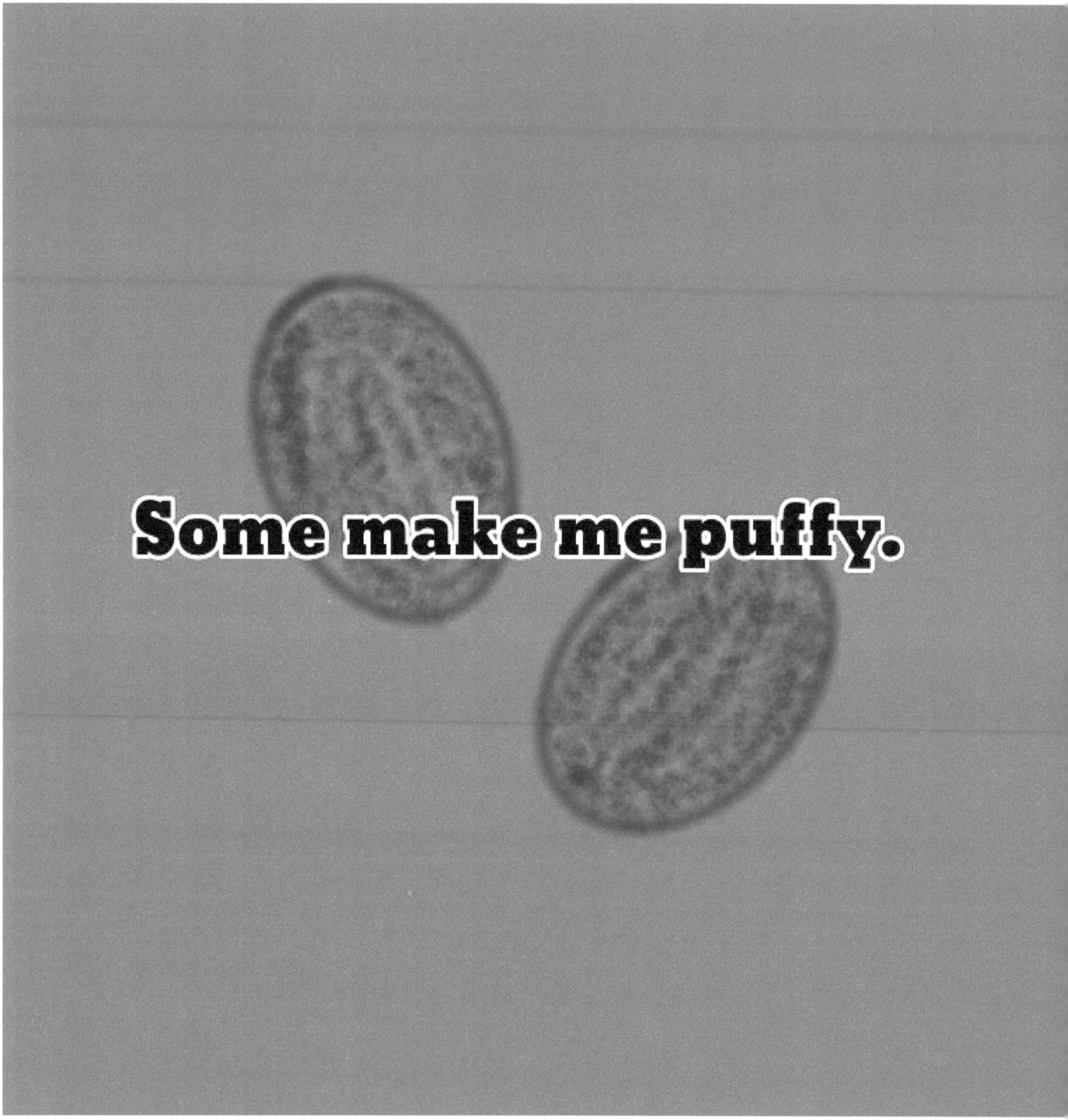

Some make me puffy.

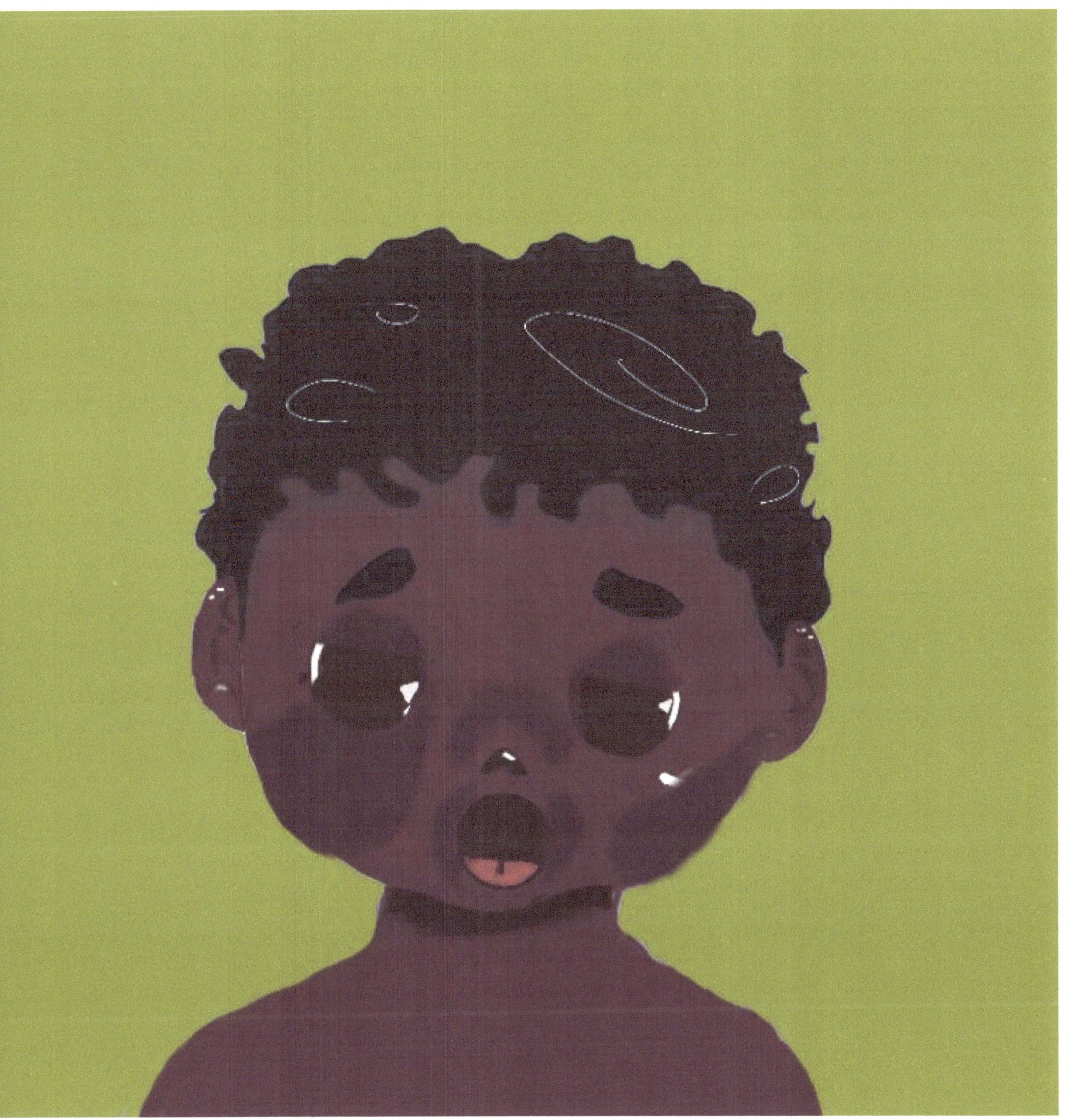

Some foods even make
my throat feel funny
and it's hard to breathe.

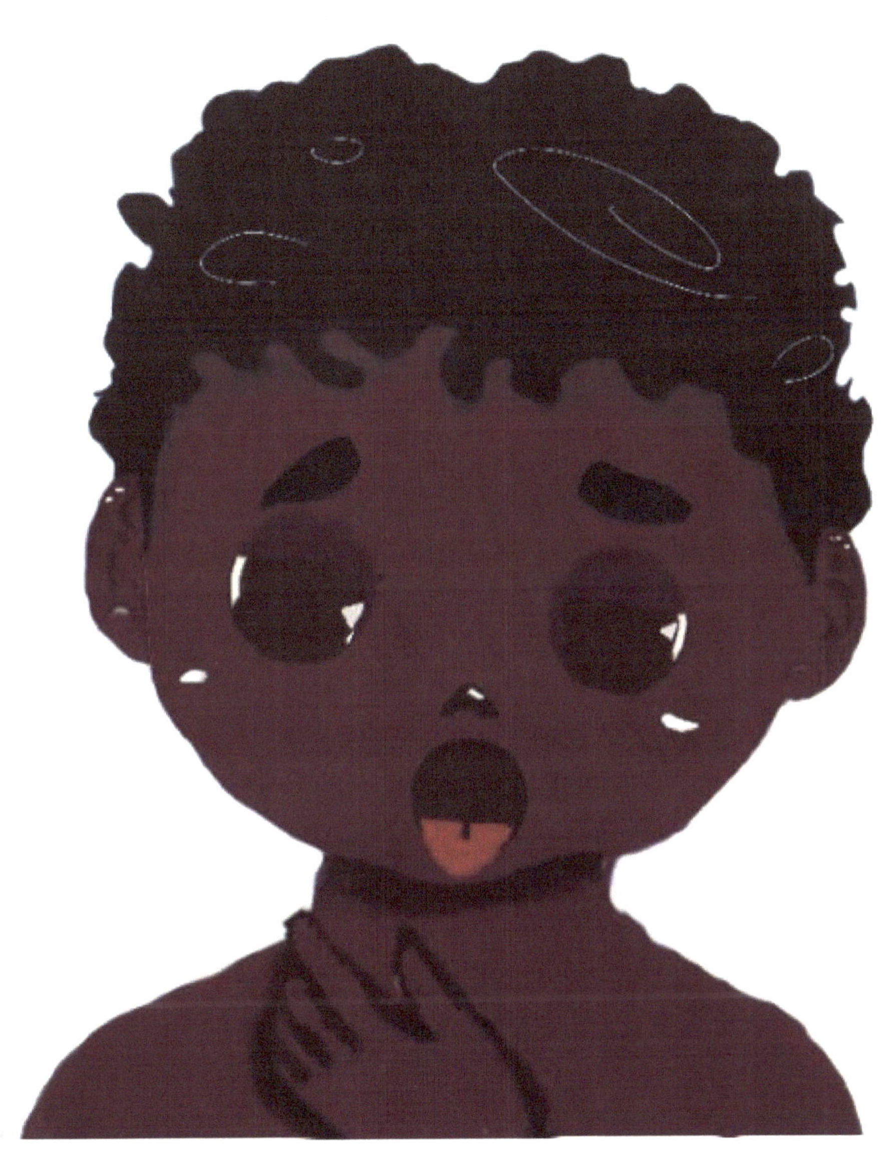

I can't eat eggs, dairy, peanuts, fish, shellfish, tree nuts, chicken or coconut.

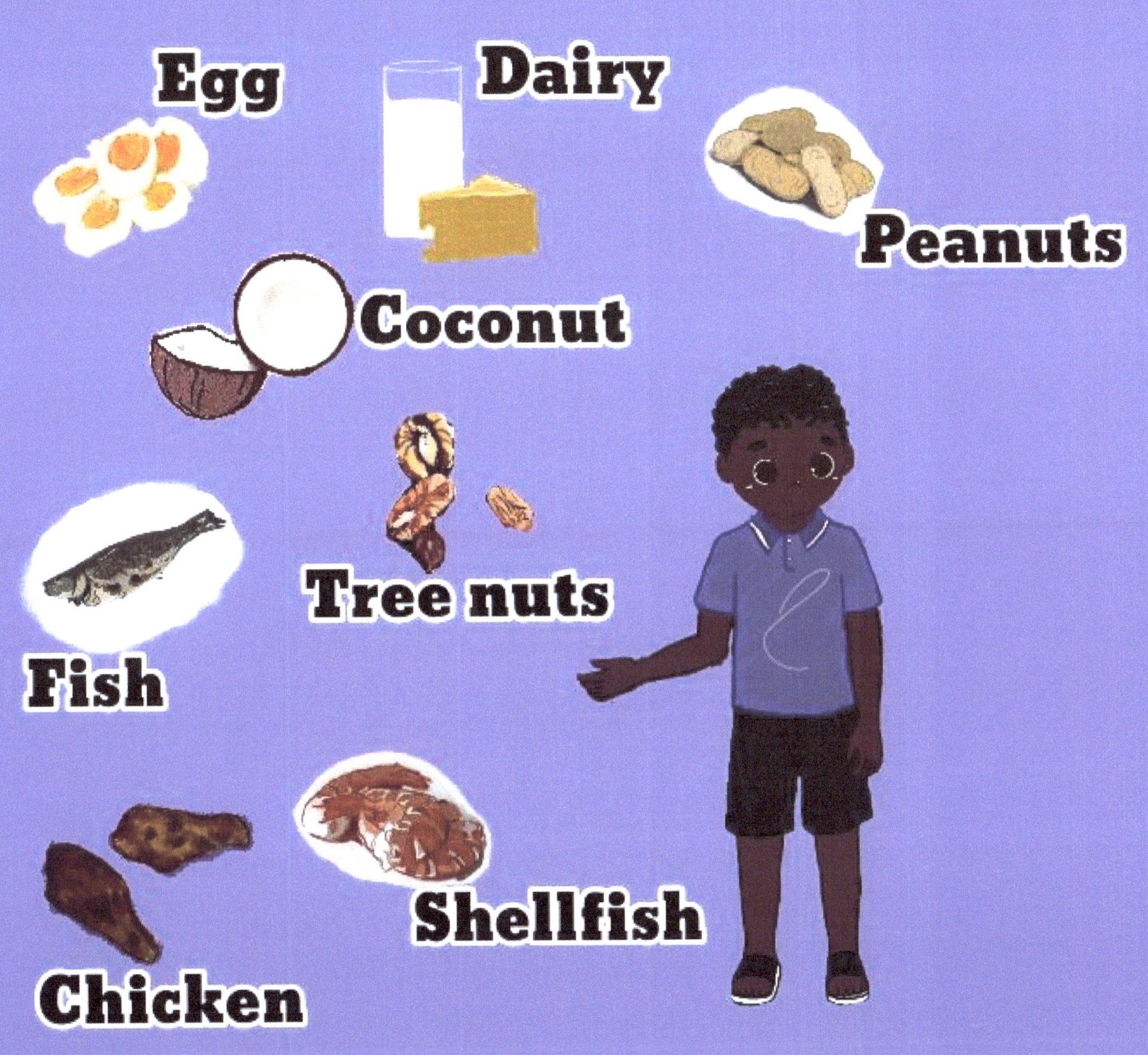

Egg
Dairy
Peanuts
Coconut
Tree nuts
Fish
Shellfish
Chicken

I know it sounds like a lot but there are a bunch of things I can eat. Foods like berries, tofu, seeds....

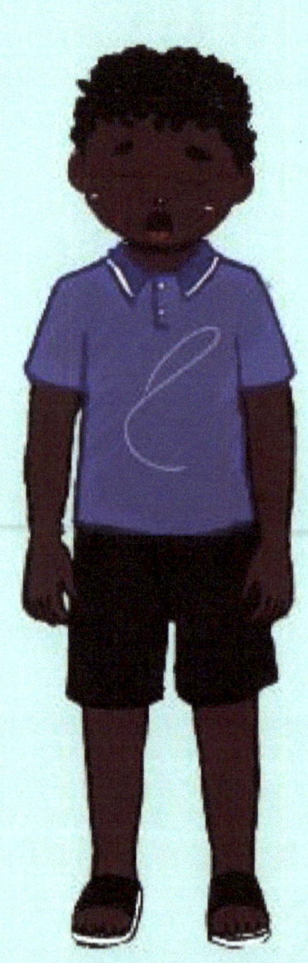

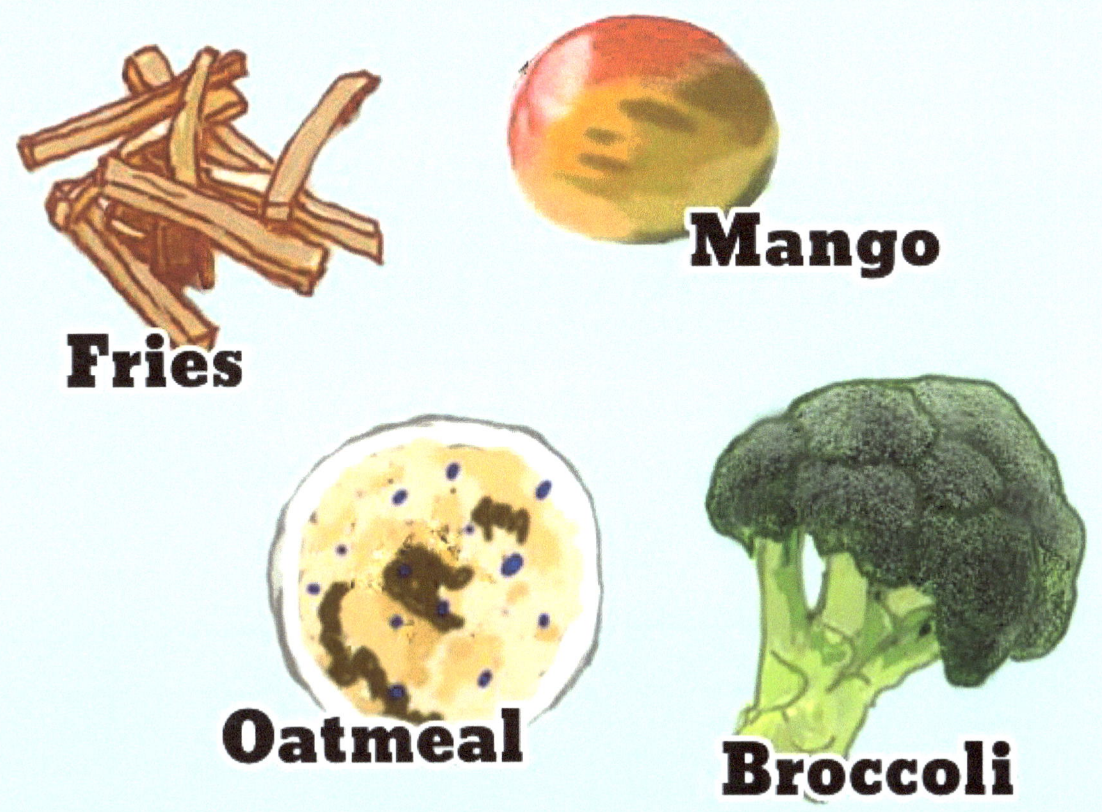

and many more.

My mom even makes me special treats like cake, cookies and candy!

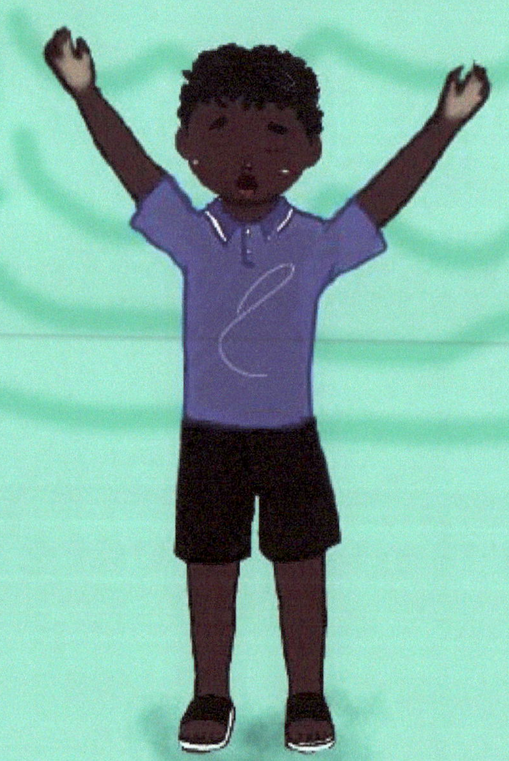

Having food allergies used to be scary for me but I know my family will take care of me. I also know how to take care of myself.

If I think I'm having an allergic reaction, I stay calm and tell a grown-up really fast.

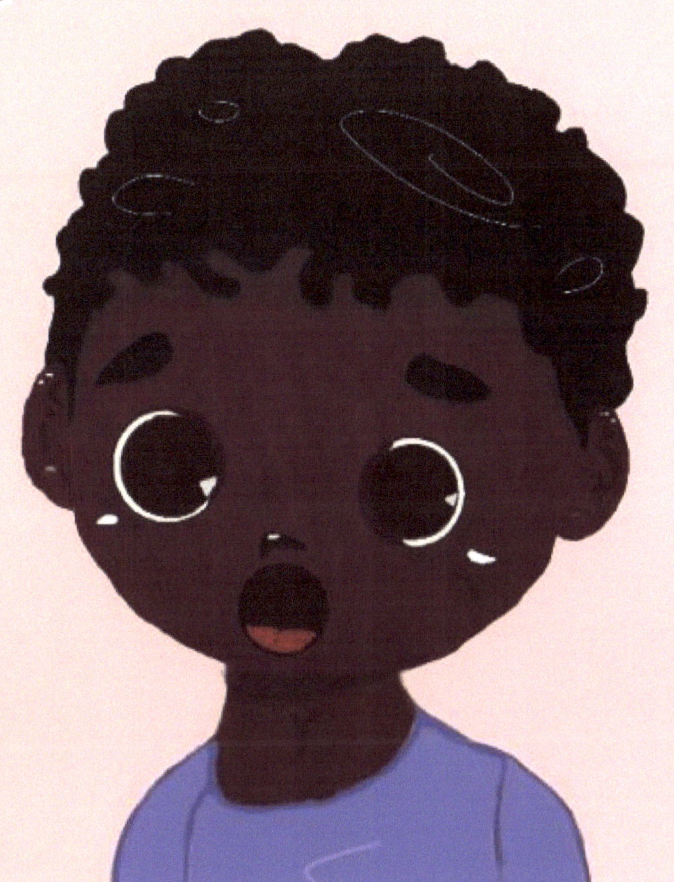
I need help!

They can help me take my medicine or use my special epi pen so that I can feel better.

EpiPen

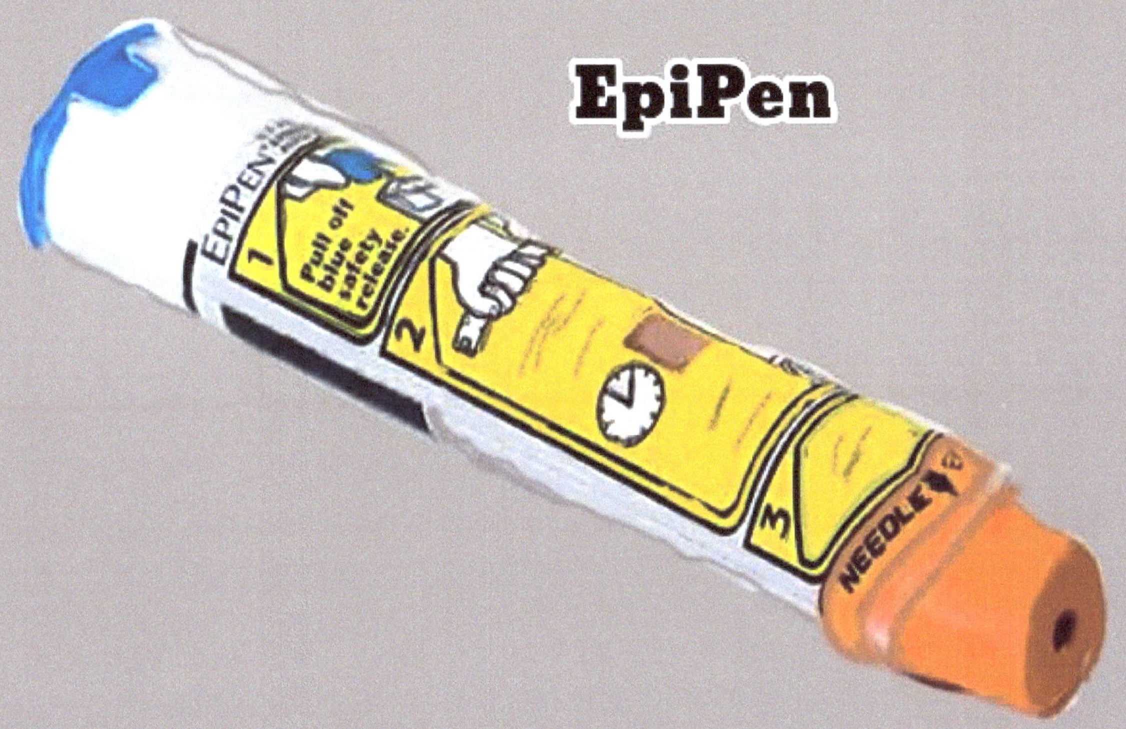

Sometimes I have to get help from my doctor too. So I Learned how to dial 911 on a phone.

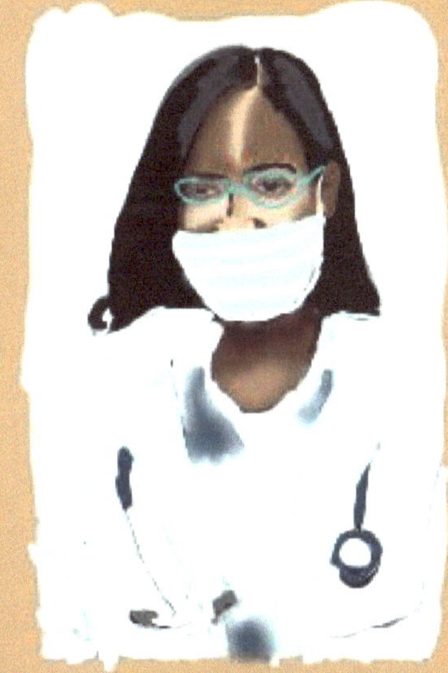

Doctor

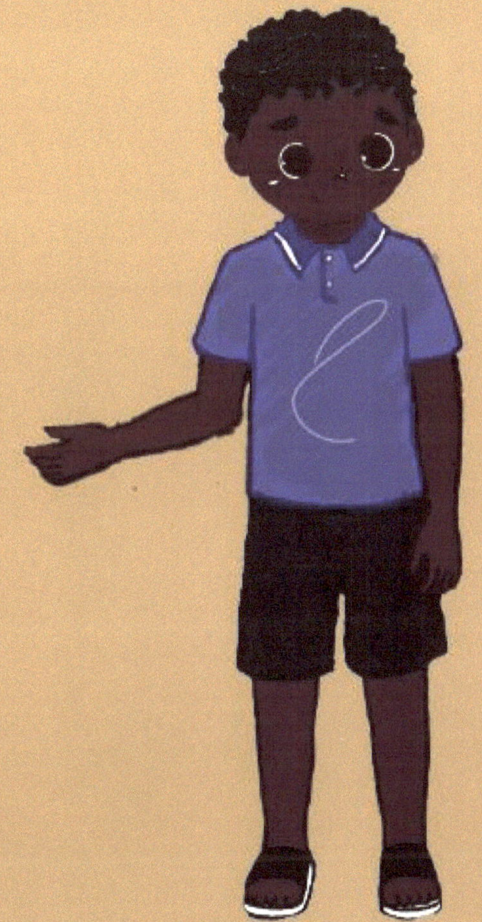

I'm not afraid of food allergies anymore because I have a safe plan.

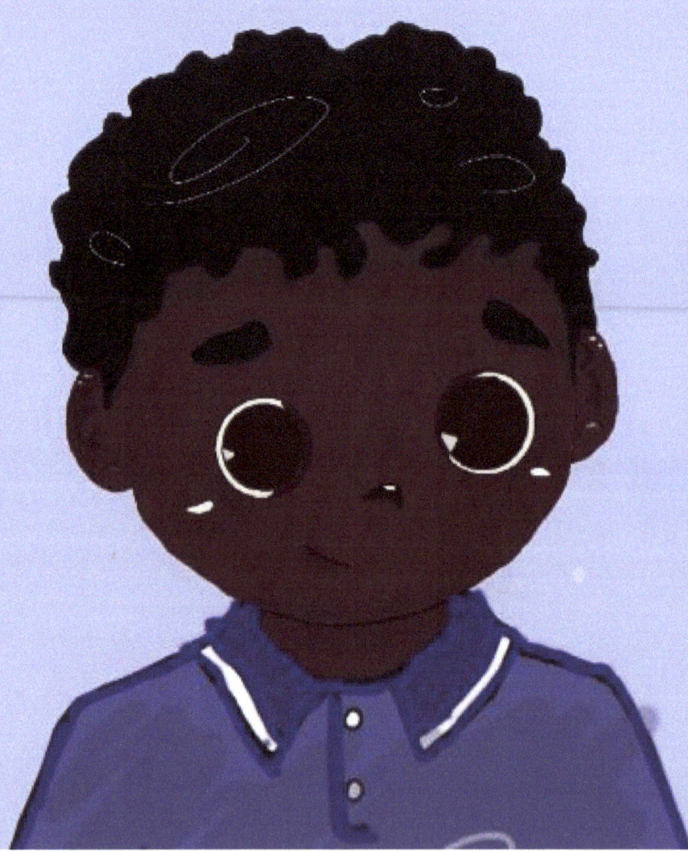

1. Stay away from foods I am allergic to.

2. Stay calm and tell a grown-up fast
if I feel sick.

3. Let a grown-up help me take my
medicine or use my epi pen.

4. Dial 911 if I need my doctor's help.

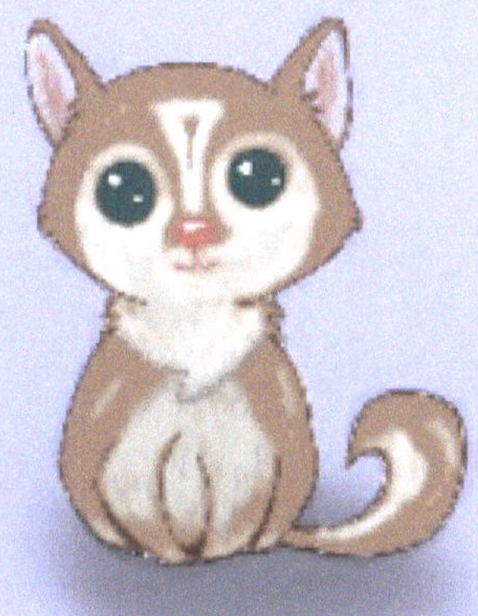

Having a safe plan helps me be brave and you can be brave too!

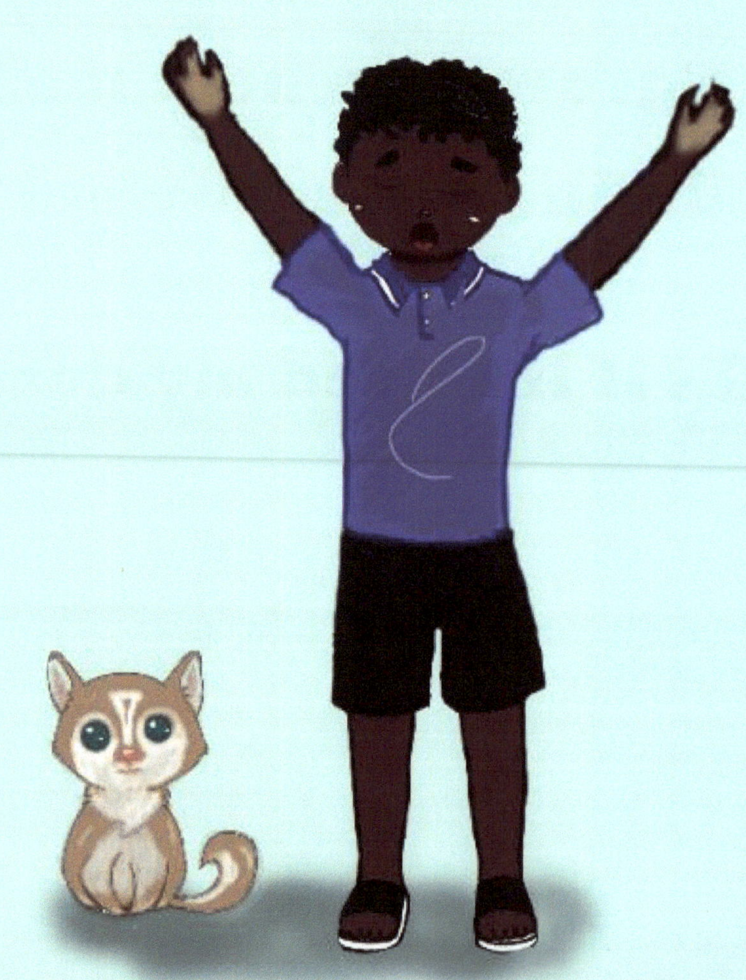

Do you have food allergies?

What are they?

What happens to your body when you eat foods you are allergic to?

Do you have a safe plan?

Have a grown-up help you make a safe plan on the next page so that you can be brave like me and star.

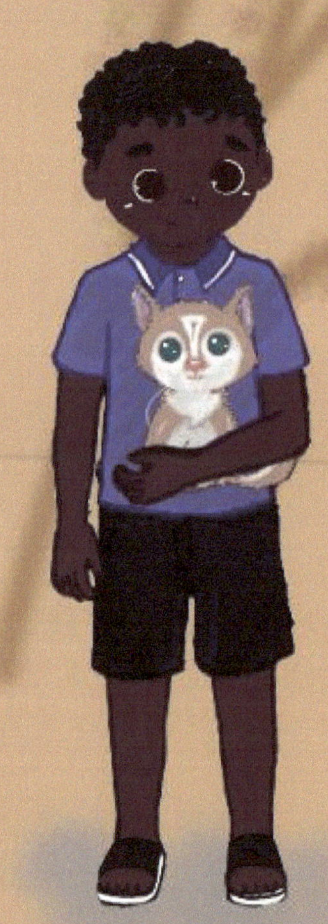

Food allergy safe plan for

Your name